# *Abiding* through the *Shadows*

## A CARETAKER'S STRUGGLE WITH GOD'S GOODNESS

ABIDING THROUGH THE SHADOWS
A CARETAKER'S STRUGGLE WITH THE GOODNESS OF GOD
published by Stronghold Press, Dallas, Texas 75238.

© 2015 by Joe and Terri Fornear
ISBN 978-0-9840113-6-0

Cover photograph © Petar Paunchev/Shutterstock.com
Book design by rhorngraphics

Unless otherwise indicated, Bible quotations are taken from The New American Standard Bible®,
© 1995 by The Lockman Foundation. Used by permission. (www.Lockman.org).


Printed in the United States of America.

**Stronghold Press**
**Dallas, Texas 75238**
www.mystronghold.org

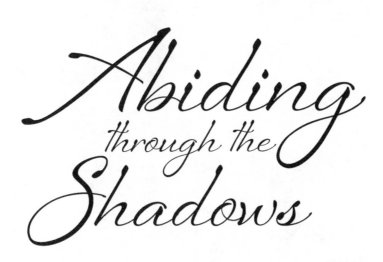

# Abiding through the Shadows

## A CARETAKER'S STRUGGLE WITH GOD'S GOODNESS

by Terri J. Fornear

STRONGHOLD
PRESS

# Contents

# Introduction

I was a pastor's wife—a person who should believe in God's love—no matter what. I should have been able to ride the storms of life with great faith and gusto. I should have been able to have an encouraging word for those in trouble.

I wish I could have been a person that always handled life right. The way people do on "Oprah"—the ones who do not even bring God into their situation. They live in the moment. They love everyone around them. They eat right, and have no regrets.

I want to share how I failed to have faith, think right, be positive or be a "good Christian" during a storm that hit our home.

My story is for the person who can't *make* himself or herself handle things right—the person who is weak, angry, and needing real GRACE. The kind of grace which says, "You do not deserve anything good because you're not doing this trial right, so let Me do it for you." The kind of grace I need.

In 2002, an uninvited visitor entered our home. I wasn't ready for it. I had not prepared myself for the mess it was about to leave. Most of all, I was not ready for this visitor to reveal "the messy home" I was already living in. The visitor's name was Stage IV Metastatic Melanoma.

God used this disease to weed out many of my religious ideas. Melanoma was the cleaning rag that God used to mop up many false beliefs about Him. It was painful though because the roots were deep and comfortable.

I needed to write my story down to remember what He did and share with my children (and others) about the grace God gave me when cancer invaded. I have shared my journey and heart honestly.

- I hope my journey helps those who deal with negativity—the people who have a difficult time seeing the positive. I hope my journey will help them come to know the grace God offers.

- I hope my journey gives courage to the fearful so that they might be real with God and allow their weaknesses to be the very tool He uses to reveal His greatness.

- I hope His unconditional love speaks loud and clear to hearts that ache to know Him without pretense.

My story is different from my husband's. He was the one who bore the physical wounds of Stage IV cancer. I am not good at relating specific details, but I will share events which left an impression on me; events that shook my relationship with God, who He is and what He is like; events which showed me the smallness of my faith. If you read both of our stories the specifics might seem a bit different. Joe and I have had a few squabbles about what happened and the timeline of events. Oh, the gift of marriage! How I love him and am so blessed he is alive so that we even get to have squabbles.

Cancer was used differently for me than for Joe. I tend to face unpleasant things with questions and anger and with a please-leave-now attitude. I tried to shoo cancer out of our home. Yet God had His timing and His purpose for each of us, which I'm still learning.

# *Part 1*

. . . . . . . . . . . . . . . . . . . . . . . . . . . . . . . . . . . . . . . . . . . . . . . . . . . . . . . . . . . . .

## My Story

*It started with …*

# Chapter 1

. . . . . . . . . . . . . . . . . . . . . . . . . . . . . . . . . . . . . . . . . . . . . . . . . . . . . . . . . . . . . . . .

## A Trip to Remember

*Now to Him who is able to do far more abundantly beyond all that we ask or think,*
*according to the power that works within us.*
*Ephesians 3:20*

The year was 2002, the year of Joe's and my 20th wedding anniversary. I wanted to celebrate—really celebrate. Plus, I was turning 49—so I was beginning the last year of my 40s. I announced to Joe how I wished to celebrate these events. I told him I didn't want flowers or dinner or even a card. He was going to have to be much more creative.

"I want a trip, a trip outside the USA. I won't settle for less." There it was—my true desire spoken out loud without guilt or false humility.

Poor Joe. He knew he could not possibly meet my expectation. We would need a miracle to pay for something so non-essential and I was being "a little" demanding. But I was hoping God could rig up my dream, my selfish dream which was not exactly a need. I was willing to wait for this dream trip. It didn't have to be on my anniversary or on my birthday. In fact I would be willing to wait all year for it.

The day after my big declaration, a dear friend called and said her boss was giving all his employees a free trip to Costa Rica, and she could take a friend. Well, that was good, but she had already invited another friend. I screamed, "What about me? I'm your friend!" I was teasing on the outside, but wishing loudly on the inside.

She came over that night with flyers and pictures and said, "Would you and Joe like to come, too? It will be totally free!" She had asked her boss and he actually said yes! It would be five days at a resort by the ocean and mountains. Amazingly, she did not even know about my desire to go on a trip "outside the USA."

Could this be real? Did God really just answer my prayer so soon?

Moments like these are scary. God had heard my prayer, my very extravagant prayer, and He answered within a couple of days. The trip was set for December 15, the day of my 49th birthday!

3

So joyfully off we went, except for one little nagging thought which I said aloud to a friend, "Do you think this trip is happening because it could be the last time Joe and I do anything fun and different, because God is tricking us and, something bad is going to happen?"

Yet, my reckless prayer was the beginning of how my relationship with God was going to take shape over the next few years. I went boldly for a miracle, for something Joe and I could not make happen with our own resources. I went to God with an honest heart without trying to manipulate Him through false humility. Just say what I want, and want what I say—and see what happens.

I was about to face deep pockets of my soul where lies about God were always affecting my daily life. They were natural to me, but they kept Him distant and unsafe.

### Mind Renewal

**Lie:** Deep down I had a belief that if something good happens then something bad must be right around the corner. God answered my prayer for a great trip, but I did not let my heart totally receive it as a love gift.

**Truth:** James 1:5 & 16: *If any of you lacks wisdom, he should ask God, who gives generously to all without finding fault, and it will be given to him. ... Don't be deceived, my dear brothers. Every good and perfect gift is from above, coming down from the Father of the heavenly lights, who does not change like shifting shadows.*

There is no "Christian Karma" in Jesus.

# Chapter 2

. . . . . . . . . . . . . . . . . . . . . . . . . . . . . . . . . . . . . . . . . . . . . . . . . . . . . . . . . . . . . . . . . .

## Bumps on the Road and Under the Arm

*Dear friends, do not be surprised at the painful trial you are suffering,*
*as though something strange were happening to you.*
1 Peter 4:12

On the Costa Rica trip, Joe seemed tired and did not want to go on any excursions. This was odd. He loves nature and crocodiles and exotic jungle animals and he passed on them all. He did not even eat all of the great food.

He kept feeling at a lump under his arm. He had a sonogram a week earlier and the tech had said the lump was lymph nodes and not a cyst, like his doctor had kept saying. When Joe called the doctor for the report, the receptionist told him the report confirmed it was just a cyst, and he could get it drained later. But it was still growing, and I think Joe was beginning to wonder if the tech was right.

We came home to a birthday cake and celebration my kids and sister had put together. It was a great trip, but there was a gnawing feeling entering in, "Lord, are you going to give us something hard to balance out this good time?"

A couple weeks later, Joe took Amy, our 15-year-old daughter, to the doctor because she was sick. While he was there he wanted to ask the doctor about the lump under his arm, as it had grown still more. The doctor left the room and came back with the sonogram report from weeks before. He must have misplaced it because he had never contacted us.

The doctors next words were, "Joe, you need to get a biopsy immediately; it looks like it is a problem in your lymph nodes."

This was the beginning of not trusting doctors. We were going to have to be very aggressive about his health and figure out what to do ourselves, a duty for which I was not equipped, but I had no choice. I felt inadequate and alone. I was a little angry at God for letting this happen to Joe. How could God let the doctor and receptionist miss this?

Time became more precious with each step we took.

5

## Mind Renewal

**Lie:** Man's mistakes have more power than God and prevent Him from working.

**Truth:** Romans 8:28: *And we know that in all things God works for the good of those who love him have been called according to his purpose.*

*Chapter 3*

. . . . . . . . . . . . . . . . . . . . . . . . . . . . . . . . . . . . . . . . . . . . . . . . . . . . .

# The Whirlwind Begins

*There they were in great fear where no fear had been.*
*Psalm 53:5*

The waiting room at the hospital was small and crowded. My church friends were kind enough to sit with me while Joe was getting surgery to have the lymph nodes biopsied. The surgeon came out to report. He was an intense man, and he did not have good news. He took me in a small room with a whiteboard. This was an interesting setup for me. God knew when I get anxious I was not good at hearing facts, so He had the doctor draw pictures. I see better than hear.

His first words were "He has metastatic cancer."

I remember saying, "What kind of cancer is that? I've heard of lots of cancers but I've never heard of that kind." He explained it's actually not a type—just saying it had spread from somewhere else to under his arm. Yet they still weren't sure where it started.

I had never been around anyone with cancer. I had been around other terminal illnesses, but not cancer. So I just sat there, puzzled and numb. I was responding more to the doctor's intensity than the verdict. He was obviously very concerned.

This was two days before Christmas 2003. We went home to wait to find out which kind of cancer Joe had.

I remember that night waking up around 3:00 a.m. A flood of fear had rushed in. I sat up in bed. The word cancer hit me hard and deep. *Is Joe going to die? What about our kids, Jesse and Amy? They are only 16 and 15 years old. They need Joe—he is the calmer parent. What about me? I need Joe. I like Joe. He's my best friend. I can't think of life without him.*

I had been married to Joe for 20 years and we also had dated for three years. He had worked out of our home so we had spent very few days apart in those 20 years.

Here it came again … that crazy concept of God which was stored deep in

7

my heart. It was gushing out in a flood of thoughts about Him. A bad thing was definitely balancing out the good.

I eventually realized that life is a mix of good and bad events. The Lord told us it would be that way and encouraged us not to be surprised. We should not judge His goodness according to our circumstances, but to look at His amazing love shown at the Cross.

**Mind Renewal**

**Lie:** God is sneaky. He gives good things just to get us ready for trials.

**Truth:** 1 Peter 4:12: *Dear friends, do not be surprised at the painful trial you are suffering, as though something strange were happening to you.*

# Chapter 4

## Waiting ... On Christmas Eve

*Behold, the virgin shall be with child and shall bear a son,*
*and they shall call his name Emmanuel, which translated means, "God with us."*
Matthew 1:23

Our family was to read a scripture on Christmas Eve at church. A nice verse that would help us focus on Christ's birth and the peacefulness of the season. I was not looking forward to all the traditions of candles, red and green bows, people dressed up in holiday clothes and all those Christmas songs. What did the holidays have to do with my "real" life now? Christmas was the farthest thing from my mind.

Yet God was so comforting. He gave me a passage for our family to share. The verses had nothing to do with Christmas, but everything to do with life.

Isaiah 46:3-4: *Listen to Me, O house of Jacob, and all the remnant of the house of Israel, you who have been borne by Me from birth and have been carried from the womb; Even to your old age I will be the same, and even to your graying years I will bear you! I have done it, and I will carry you; and I will bear you and I will deliver you.*

I stood strong sharing these verses which said He would bear us up in our graying years. He would deliver us. This Child that was born on Christmas was going to show me the way of deliverance.

**Mind Renewal**

**Lie:** Jesus' birth really isn't relevant to my life today. Is Jesus God, and if He is, how does that make a difference in my life—now?

9

**Truth:** Ephesians 1:18-21: *I pray also that the eyes of your heart may be enlightened in order that you may know the hope to which he has called you, the riches of his glorious inheritance in the saints, and his incomparably great power for us who believe. That power is like the working of his mighty strength, which he exerted in Christ when he raised him from the dead and seated him at his right hand in the heavenly realms, far above all rule and authority, power and dominion, and every title that can be given, not only in the present age but also in the one to come.*

I needed my eyes opened!

# Chapter 5

. . . . . . . . . . . . . . . . . . . . . . . . . . . . . . . . . . . . . . . . . . . . . . . . . . . . . . . . . .

# Still WAITING

*For the inhabitant of Maroth becomes weak waiting for good.*
*Micah 1:12*

Joe's diagnosis changed three times, ending with metastatic melanoma. I mention metastatic, because people would tell me they once had melanoma —a skin spot removed. Yet Joe never even had a spot on his skin. It went directly to his lymph nodes, so it was metastatic because it spread past the skin. This was one of those unanswerable questions we kept asking. How could he catch it in time if he never had a skin lesion?

Waiting for the name of the cancer was the first obstacle over which I became very anxious. It seemed to me the sooner we knew the sooner we could stop it. Yet the timing was so out of our hands. The passing of so much time felt like a death sentence.

Joe needed a second surgery to remove the remainder of the lymph nodes under his arm. He was scheduled to have surgery the following week. Hopefully, we would then be free of this monster.

After his surgery, the doctor took me into the little room again to tell me some good news and some bad news. First, he felt he got all of the remainder of the cancer under Joe's arm. But the results of a new PET scan and biopsy showed a cancer lesion in his stomach. The melanoma was either spreading quickly, or they had found the source of the cancer—the primary—in his stomach.

We had been hoping for a different kind of cancer than melanoma. After researching stomach cancer on the internet, we found there was a low side effect pill which had a great record of stopping it. I am not sure I was reading all the right information, but one thing was clear—stomach cancer had way better statistics than melanoma. If this was Stage IV melanoma, there was only a six percent chance of any treatment working.

Our family was already dealing with metastatic melanoma. In fact Joe's dad, who lived far from Dallas in Pittsburgh, had just been diagnosed with Stage IV melanoma and given a few months. He was getting worse and Joe wanted to go see him. We had been planning to go at Christmas, however, our uninvited visitor would not allow us to leave.

> **Mind Renewal**
>
> **Lie:** Understanding what is happening in my life will give me the power to control it. Knowledge can make everything bad go away!
>
> **Truth:** Proverbs 3:5-7: *Trust in the LORD with all your heart and lean not on your own understanding; in all your ways acknowledge Him, and He will make your paths straight. Do not be wise in your own eyes.*

# Chapter 6

. . . . . . . . . . . . . . . . . . . . . . . . . . . . . . . . . . . . . . . . . . . . . . . . . . . . . . . . . . .

## Two Surgeries, Two Cuts: The Invisible Knife

*When I pondered to understand this, it was troublesome in my sight.*
*Psalms 73:16*

The morning of Joe's stomach surgery I was alone in the waiting room except for an older man and his daughter waiting for his wife to come out of surgery. Because it was so quiet, I could not help overhearing them. The man said, "I dread this disease. Every time they go into get some out, it seems to spread further and further. Melanoma has no end."

Anxiety swelled up in my heart. They had no idea I was waiting for Joe to come out of surgery for the same disease. This man's wife was in her 70s, so I reasoned, perhaps they were preparing to let her go. But Joe was in his 40s. *He has two kids. He needs to live!*

Moments like these just reveal the fear in my heart. I can entertain every wrong thing that can possibly happen, play it out, and try to solve it. I couldn't even tell you if others entered the room. I was alone and trying to live my life years down the road.

I had not put on the shield of faith. I was caught off guard, not ready for the intensity of that battle in the waiting room. The roaring lion had been waiting for this opportunity, roaring loud and clear that my children and I would never make it.

While Joe's stomach was being cut, I was being "cut" in my heart. Nobody saw it happening. There was no blood. No doctor was going to tell my loved ones how I was recovering. These battles are only seen in the invisible world where spiritual battles are fought over our beliefs in God. Is He good no matter what? Can we trust Him to provide and care for us in the future? Will He carry me through the next hour? Maybe He'll notice how upset I am and fix everything.

The doctor came out and told me he believed he got it all, but we needed to get a plan that kills the smallest cells of melanoma. He was going to turn us over to an oncologist now. He hoped it all would turn out okay.

Time felt like our greatest enemy and our oncologist did not seem in a hurry to get rolling. We waited for an appointment.

**Mind Renewal**

**Lie:** Anxiety and worry will stop God from fixing my problem. But I can't stop worrying so maybe if I really worry, God will fix my problem. I can manipulate God through worry.

**Truth:** Matthew 6:27: *Who of you by worrying can add a single hour to his life?*

# Chapter 7

· · · · · · · · · · · · · · · · · · · · · · · · · · · · · · · · · · · · · · · · · · · · · · · · · · · · · · · · ·

## He Speaks In the Storm

*Thus the LORD used to speak to Moses face to face,*
*just as a man speaks to his friend.*
*Exodus 33:11*

I love God's Word. He speaks directly into my heart to the fears which seem so loud. The voice of the God of the universe of which I knew so little became more real to me. I am but a speck on this planet, yet He wanted to teach me His voice and heart as if I were the only one alive. He wanted me to let go of the lies I had kept in my heart about Him.

He wanted my friendship. He made John 15:15 come alive.

*No longer do I call you slaves, for the slave does not know what his master is doing. But I called you friends. For all the things that I have heard from My Father I have made known to you.*

He wanted me to know He was going to walk us through this, each specific step. I needed to know He was on my side. The lies I created about Him needed to be exchanged for the truth about Him. Truth always takes me back to His cross.

I think lies were my safeguard against really letting Him have my life. I wanted control of the things I love—my family, friends, church, etc. As if I could keep them safe and untouched from evil and death. After all, God allows bad things to happen to everyone. So how could I trust Him?

He spoke to me through Proverbs 3:5-6, "Trust me wholeheartedly, in every corner of your life. Recognize that I am in charge to make your path smooth. I will take care of each obstacle in the trial ahead."

His Word began touching the very lies I held onto for safety. Reading His Word was no longer an activity I did to please Him. I realized at times I had used Bible reading like a rabbit's foot. If I started my day off reading the Bible, good things would happen. He wanted to change this approach to His Word. He wanted me to know Him as the *life source* to live by each day. His Word became *life* to me. It gave me a peace that was above reason and a power that showed up when I was weak. It was my daily bread to live on. I could let go of my fears and be real with Him because He didn't seem threatened by my lack of faith in His goodness. He just wanted to have a chance to love me and shed light into the shadows of my fears. Hearing His voice helped me to wait in peace.

The stomach tumor was sent to a stomach specialist at the University of Washington, still hoping it would be a strain of stomach cancer. But we got a "positive" report—positive for melanoma. Because of its reputation, knowing the name only brought more fear. Yet God reminded me He was in charge of melanoma too and He was bigger than statistics.

---

### Mind Renewal

**Lie:** My false concept of God prevents God from loving and showing Himself to me.

**Truth:** Romans 3:4-5: *What if some did not have faith? Will their lack of faith nullify God's faithfulness? Not at all! Let God be true, and every man a liar.*

---

## Chapter 8

......................................................................

# A Sprout of Hope

*For there is hope for a tree;*
*When it is cut down, that it will sprout again,*
*and its shoots will not fail.*
*Job 14:7*

Joe missed visiting his dad at Christmas because of the biopsy surgeries under his arm. Then in late January of 2003, he had the stomach surgery. During recovery, he asked the doctor if he thought he could travel to Pittsburgh to see his dad who was getting worse. I know Joe wanted to share the gospel with his dad so that he was clear on the way to heaven (through faith in Jesus alone). Yet I remember Joe lying in the hospital bed in a lot of pain. The doctor was sitting on one side of the bed and I on the other. I kept staring at the doctor, hoping he saw my concerns. I wanted him to say "No, take care of yourself first."

Now Joe, being a pastor, had often made me feel like others were first. I wondered if as a pastor he thought he was paid to think of others first. The non-paid Christian did not have to give when there was nothing more to give. It wasn't their profession. Yet Joe would want to travel, especially to see his dad, even if it was the last thing he did.

As I sat across from the doctor, he could read me pretty well. He encouraged Joe not to go right away. He suggested giving himself a week or two to recover. Joe submitted to that idea, but with a lot of frustration.

Soon the decision to travel or not became even more intense. Joe's dad died a few days later, the day Joe was to be released from the hospital. The funeral would be in just four days. Thankfully, Joe knew there was no way he could travel that soon. Still, this was Joe's lowest point so far. The sadness of not being able to visit his dad or even go to his funeral made his recovery even harder and the reality of this disease more real. His dad's passing scared me too.

When we visited the oncologist whom the surgeon referred, he recommended Interleukin 2 (Il-2), Joe's best hope for beating this cancer. He said it would give him a 6% chance of living —not much, but at least it was a sprout.

The doctor said the best hospital for this treatment was out of town and just happened to be in Pittsburgh where Joe's dad had just passed. So Joe planned to go for the first three weeks of the treatment as he could be with his family and stay with his mother. This gave him opportunity to grieve his dad's death with his family. God knew the right time. Later, Joe's sister said it was good that he did not see his dad because his dad's battle was painful to watch. Since Joe was dealing with the same cancer, it could have added more discouragement and fear.

Joe traveled alone and the kids and I stayed in Dallas with plans for periodic visits. I felt out of control already, and now we wouldn't even be together.

### Mind Renewal

**Lie:** Joe's dad died of melanoma; therefore Joe is definitely going to die of melanoma as well.

**Truth:** Psalm 139:16: *Your eyes saw my unformed body. All the days ordained for me were written in your book before one of them came to be.*

## Chapter 9

................................................................

# Angels Watching Over Them

*For I have come to have much joy and comfort in your love,*
*because the hearts of the saints have been refreshed through you, brother.*
*Philemon 1:7*

Fighting the cancer took a lot of time, keeping up with all of the treatments, appointments and complications. I began to be very concerned how all of this would impact the kids. I could see the gaps forming in what we were giving compared to what I thought they needed.

Jesse was 16 at the time. He was a quiet kid, but very in tune to what was going on around him. His quiet and steady faith gave him a strength that allowed him to stand alone.

Amy was 15. She has a simple, concrete faith that makes others chuckle ... and wonder.

We sat them down and proceeded to share about our battle. Jesse took a long, deep breath before we even opened our mouth. He heard every phone conversation, every whisper out of our mouths.

"You both realize I am sick," said Joe. "This disease is called melanoma—a cancerous skin disease. The same one Grandpa had. People die with it. But we are going to pray for a miracle."

Jesse's response was quiet but strong. "But Dad, not everybody dies from cancer."

Amy's response was excitement. "God is going to do something great."

Then we prayed and said, "That's all for now." I was crying the whole time. My family thinks I am too emotional anyway because I am Italian. I think they were more interested in keeping me comforted than sharing their own fears at the time. Their feelings came out in brief comments and at odd times throughout the ordeal. They felt safest to share when I was hopeful.

It was then that the hands and feet of the body of Christ came alongside us and held them up with their kindness. People of whom we expected little came through in big ways. God choose our comforters and the kid's comforters as well.

A father in our church was taking his son on a father/child camp for a week in the mountains of Colorado. Joe could not go, so this friend invited Amy to be his temporary daughter for the week. This excited Amy and it filled our hearts with God's love and care in a big way.

When she came back it was the first time she shared her feelings about Joe's ordeal. I think getting away allowed her to face and process what was happening without worrying about being "negative."

She also had a basketball coach who took her under his wing. He was a Christian and they shared the Lord a lot together. He invited her to go on a sports mission trip to China with a team in the summer—a life-changing experience for her. She spent three weeks watching him and his fiancée keep Christ first in their relationship. This gave her a glimpse of the type of guy with whom she would eventually want to share life. We did not have to sit Amy down and teach her about looking for the right guy. The Lord showed her up close what a brother looks like when he is dating a woman with God's goals for their relationship.

Jesse's support came in different ways. His sensitive heart always made me want to protect him more. Yet he was more level-headed and dependable than I thought. He would do anything we asked. I just hated asking him to do much because I just wanted him to be a normal 16-year-old. I wanted him to disagree with me and yell and do things that showed he did not have to take care of me. I guess I had bought into our culture's idea that a teenager needs to be rebellious in order to find himself and be independent. Jesse was clay in our hands, but our hands were pretty full. So I often feared he was left too much to himself. It was great when a family paid his way to a summer camp ministry which definitely encouraged him.

He also spent a lot of time with another family with whom we had been long time friends. Their son and Jesse went to elementary school together. This family was another one of those families with the gift of mercy who often jumped in to help when we were at our bottom. The mom had a simple faith. It was exactly what I needed at the time. Once she went with me to Baylor Medical Center to check out clinical trials if we ran out of standard options. Whenever the nurses or doctor sounded negative about Joe's situation and I got fearful, she would just laugh and act like it did not matter what they said. I would laugh at her because she made it seem so simple. At times it made melanoma feel like a piece of bad candy which I could just throw away. I really needed that.

Our youth pastor at the time was also a real gift. He was older than most youth pastors and had a mature relationship with Jesus. He would simply ask

Jesse how he was doing and let him know he cared. He put no pressure on him to pour out his feelings. I think his steady love for the Lord gave Jesse a security with God which spoke louder than words. He was a blessing to our family.

All of this "outside" help was so against all of my Christian rules of parenting. I had let James Dobson down. As a parent, I was not doing the job which God had given to me. Little did I know that God had been parenting the kids all along, even through our inabilities, inadequacies and weaknesses.

Even today, I've had to continually trust God to fill any gaps of nurture which Joe and I could not personally provide at that time. It's funny how life happens and our children have their own story to form their own relationship with God.

---

**Mind Renewal**

**Lie:** It was entirely up to Joe and me to make sure we parented our children through trials correctly so that they would be okay.

**Truth:** Ephesians 2:10: *For we are God's workmanship, created in Christ Jesus to do good works, which God prepared in advance for us to do.*

---

God has our kid's lives worked out. Along with the cancer, my faults, inadequacies and failures are some of the tools He used and still uses to bring about His purposes for them.

# Chapter 10

. . . . . . . . . . . . . . . . . . . . . . . . . . . . . . . . . . . . . . . . . . . . . . . . . . . . . . .

## Separation's Pain

*Precious in the sight of the LORD Is the death of His godly ones.*
*Psalm 116:15*

When Joe went to Pittsburgh for Il-2, I was torn. I wanted to be with him, but the kids needed to finish school and keep things "normal." I thought we could manage three weeks apart, but the three weeks turned into seven. I realized it was possible that Joe might die in Pittsburgh.

Here again the body of Christ gave to our family. A family in the neighborhood who was involved in Young Life came with a dinner and a heart which heard my need to be with Joe. They offered to buy me a round trip ticket to Pittsburgh to spend a weekend with Joe.

I went to see him, but it was a really difficult time. Because of the roughness of the treatment, he seemed so alone, even though his family was there. His brothers and sisters stayed with him at night. His mom had to watch him battle with the same disease which took her husband just weeks earlier. They were all grieving his father's death. Joe felt bad he was such a burden they had to keep bearing.

I tended to keep things to myself even when lots of people were around. Yet I remember the day I was to return to Dallas, standing in the kitchen at five in the morning crying and unloading on his brother who was my chauffeur all week. "I do not want to leave, I can't leave." I wanted my children to be with us. Was I to have separation from Joe, or from the kids? Torn again.

As I rode to the airport, I heard the Shepherd's voice, "Do you feel that separation? That's how I feel with my children who are on earth. I am working in all generations and time to bring MY family together. The Christian world calls this the end times. I call it the beginning of the greatest family reunion in all eternity. I do delight in the death of my kids because I get to see them face to face."

Psalm 116:15 says, "Precious in the sight of the LORD is the death of His godly ones."

This verse reminded me He hated death so much that He built a bridge through His Son to eliminate its consequence. He never intended for this thing called death to enter His creation. He hated death and did something about it when He asked His Son to deal with it on the cross. Something He did not create He had to eliminate.

Yet Jesus said He was the resurrection and life and He defeated death. There is so much in what He said which I cannot grasp, but I realized at that moment with our battle with death He wanted me to see He hated it more than I hated it. He did not like separation either. He gave up His Son for this enemy.

Psalm 116:15 made sense for the first time. I realized if Joe lived, God was letting go of seeing him face-to-face and giving us more time with him. He was willing to be physically separated longer from Him during this dot in time. I really can't imagine what it will be like to see Him face to face, but He is love, so it's bound to be good!

I went home to Dallas and gathered the kids and came right back to Pittsburgh. Fortunately it was spring break. Once more someone bought our tickets to do this—Joe's cousin this time. When I think of the practical needs of families fighting cancer, I think of travel costs, as so many of the best trials require travel. We were blessed to have Joe's family in Pittsburgh, but many don't know anyone in the city they must go for treatment. Many have no money to take their children during treatment. Some pass away in hospitals miles from their home.

Separation is a part of life we have to face in this life and certainly in the deaths of loved ones. Yet God surely understands our feelings of separation-anxiety. I'm sure that is why He constantly reminds us He will never leave or forsake us.

### Mind Renewal

**Lie:** God doesn't really care how death and separation hurts people.

**Truth:** 2 Corinthians 1:9-10: *Indeed, in our hearts we felt the sentence of death. But this happened that we might not rely on ourselves but on God, who raises the dead. He has delivered us from such a deadly peril, and he will deliver us. On him we have set our hope that he will continue to deliver us.*

# Chapter 11

## THE PROMISE

····································································

*And you brethren, like Isaac, are children of promise.*
*Galatians 4:28*

This was the beginning of my real journey of faith. The longest Joe and I had ever been separated was when he went on a two-week mission trip to the Middle East. Since he works out of our home we are used to being together 24/7 (which has given us moments of craziness). But this was our first separation without an end-date. I was alone with God. I needed to hear from Him for myself. I needed to seek Him for direction and faith. How did He want me to pray? Was I to claim healing like I saw on TV? Was my faith going to be what healed Joe? Why did God heal some Christians and not others?

I cried out to Him with ears to hear. I was in our bed alone and having trouble sleeping. The turning point for me was during the second week of our separation. That night I had finally gone to sleep, but woke up around 3 a.m. which seemed to be my magic hour. John 15:7 was on my mind.

*If you abide in Me and My words abide in you ask whatever you wish and it will be done for you.*

I had this simple lightness of heart. I remember laughing at God and asked Him, "Are You saying I can ask *whatever* I wish and You will give it to me?" Well, I am not a stupid person so I remember getting right to the point with Him. "Then I am going to ask You to let Joe be completely healed of Stage IV melanoma." I felt like I had to be clear with my wish because it was a clear and simple verse. It was such a childlike dialogue. I felt foolish, but very brave.

I had complete assurance that God was going to answer ... just like He had answered my Costa Rica trip prayer. That night I slept like I had not slept for months. I had so much peace and assurance.

Yet when I woke up the next morning, I thought I should read the verse in context in case there was a great big "but" or something else I had missed which would show I was not interpreting the verse correctly.

As I read it I read all the way to verse 16, I realized He was saying it to me twice!

*Did I not say that whatever you ask of the Father in My name, I will give you?*

All I could say was, "Okay, okay, I BELIEVE YOU. And I receive from YOU." Right then I had confidence He was going to heal Joe completely.

Faith is not easy. No matter how assured I felt at that time, I was going to have to offer His promise back to Him.

---

**Mind Renewal**

**Lie:** I can't trust myself to hear God.

**Truth:** John 15:15: *I no longer call you servants, because a servant does not know his master's business. Instead, I have called you friends, for everything that I learned from my Father I have made known to you.*

---

# Chapter 12

## Promise Breaker?

*All these died in faith, without receiving the promises, but having seen them and having welcomed them from a distance, and having confessed that they were strangers and exiles on the earth.*
*Hebrews 11:13*

Joe returned from Pittsburgh with a body full of melanoma having used up his best human chance of receiving healing. The Interleukin-2 did not work. Cancer had spread to his lung, kidney and pancreas—a total of 13 different spots. He could not eat because of the pain in his pancreas and had lost over 60 pounds. He could barely walk because cancer was in his pelvis. He was dying.

When I saw his suffering and that he wanted to go, I stood before God like a crazy lady and in anger said these words:

*"All right, You are God; You can do whatever You wish, but do not ask me to pray what I wish and then act like You are going to keep Your promise. You can change Your mind. You can do whatever You want. You are God whether you keep Your promise or not. I will believe in You. I will follow You. Please keep my heart from being mad at You. I can't seem to work that out of me. And yes, I am mad at You and I do not like You and I am sorry for that. I am sorry that I am not the perfect little Christian handling this in the right way. You seem mean to me and like You are a liar, but I have nowhere else to go."*

I could not use my goodness, my Christianity, or my right thinking to manipulate God to keep the promise which I thought He gave to me. I had come to the end of my good behavior ... and my faith.

I was wondering if I was like one of those people in Hebrews chapter 11. I was going to watch Joe die without receiving the promise God gave me. These kinds of struggles are between God and the heart. Somehow He got my heart to let go and cling to Him as my life. I was walking out a faith that was truly without sight. I was left with God's love—wrapped in letting go of His Son—a love that faced death with pain and loneliness. He was letting me feel the death of the cross. It appeared that God had lost and the enemy had won at the cross.

Each day as I saw Joe get thinner and cry from pain I felt like a nail was stabbing my heart. All I could do was watch and wonder where all that "God love" was.

No resurrection in sight.

---

**Mind Renewal**

**Lie:** God doesn't keep His promises to me. God changes His promises.

**Truth:** 2 Corinthians 1:20: *For no matter how many promises God has made, they are "Yes" in Christ. And so through him the "Amen" is spoken by us to the glory of God.*

---

# Chapter 13

· · · · · · · · · · · · · · · · · · · · · · · · · · · · · · · · · · · · · · · · · · · · · · · · · · ·

## Thy Will Be Done

*Thy will be done on earth as it is in Heaven.*
*Matthew 6:10*

One of my prayers during this time was The Lord's Prayer. Having been raised Catholic, I called it "The Our Father." I was familiar with it as part of the rosary and we also had to pray it as part of our penance after confessing sins. I was also raised Lutheran because of my mom's side of the family, and we recited it in our weekly services. I think I had used it like a rabbit's foot of good luck—until this disease happened.

People kept saying to me, "God's will be done." Since Jesus said it in the Garden of Gethsemane and taught us to pray it in The Our Father I didn't think I could argue.

Yet one morning as I was reading The Our Father in Matthew, I saw the phrase after "Thy will be done." It said, "Thy will be done—*on earth as it is in heaven.*" I remember talking back to Him in a sarcastic way. "Is melanoma in heaven?" Here again my literalism was causing some real questioning. Of course, the answer is no. Melanoma is not in heaven; there is no disease in heaven.

I could sense His same smile when He said, "Ask whatever you wish…" He whispered in my spirit, "Ask Me to bring heaven to earth for you." I began praying, "Thy will be done as it is in heaven." Whenever someone would say, "You need to want God's will more than anything," I told them I *did* want God's will more than anything. I wanted heaven to come to earth.

Now I don't want to write a theological book on prayer. I guess I do not care if anyone else thinks I interpreted these verses right. I just sensed I had some ground to go boldly to the throne of grace and ask for melanoma to be gone. So I did. I now had a shield around me that would extinguish the fiery arrows of doubt around those Thy-will-be-done prayers. At first, I began holding it up quietly as I heard others pray. I would say, "As it is in heaven, Father, as it is in heaven—where Jesus sits next to You with dried blood on His hands interceding for us saying 'It is finished. By My stripes Joe has been healed.'"

28

Oh how I love hearing our Father's voice and direction over the voices of dark spiritual authorities and even well-meaning people. Together, Jesus and I were piercing the darkness in my world with weapons of heaven.

---

**Mind Renewal**

**Lie:** His will is always different than mine; that's why I have to end every prayer that way—with "but Thy will be done."

**Truth:** John 15:7-9: *If you abide in Me, and My words abide in you, ask whatever you wish, and it will be done for you. My Father is glorified by this, that you bear much fruit, and so prove to be My disciples. Just as the Father has loved Me, I have also loved you; abide in My love.*

---

God wants to hear my "wishes." I don't have to pretend I won't hurt if I don't get what I want. He can keep me from bitterness if I am honest with Him.

# Chapter 14

## A Glimmer of Light

*For He will give His angels charge concerning you, to guard you in all your ways.*
*Psalm 91:11*

A friend knew the daughter of a woman from her "Moms in Touch" group who had lived 11 years with Stage IV melanoma. I just knew I needed to talk to that family.

The woman's husband was as much a melanoma fighter as her. He had done extensive research on melanoma. In fact, it was clear he helped keep his wife alive for such a long time.

Here was my angel. Here was the light which was going to lead us step-by-step to experience God's promise. When I asked him what doctors he thought were the best for melanoma, he told us about a Jewish doctor with a lot of heart and another who did high-beam guided radiation.

We immediately made appointments to see both of these doctors. Joe was so sick by the time we got to the oncologist that he just wanted to relieve Joe's pain and keep him comfortable. Eventually, he told Joe to get his house in order because he only had days to live. Joe's response was to tell the doctor that he was dying too. Joe asked if he knew whether or not he was going to heaven. They had a great two-hour talk about God, Jesus, and what real life is all about. He is a God-fearing man who we pray will take Jesus as his Savior before he dies.

This oncologist put Joe on TPN which is basically intravenous nutrition. He was on it for around six weeks. Because he couldn't eat anything, we believe this was one of the tools God used to save Joe's life. As we hear the stories of other late stage cancer patients we realize not many doctors offer this choice because they think it just prolongs the inevitable. So we are very thankful our doctor ordered this, because we had never even heard of TPN. It bought us time for our next steps.

The doctor wanted Joe to be admitted immediately to the hospital to get stabilized. While there, he discussed a chemotherapy cocktail which he said offered almost no chance of working and would cause Joe to be miserable from the side effects. Since the strong chemo could also kill him, the doctor did not recommend it at all. He was trying to help Joe get prepared to die, but we thought if he was going to die anyway, we might as well try this chemo.

One evening I asked the doctor when we were going to start the chemo. So he scheduled the first round to be given while Joe was still in the hospital. It was awful. He had a terrible reaction and almost died on the spot of a heart problem.

Interestingly though, God had allowed two of his many tumors to grow right under the skin on Joe's collar bone. We could feel them and watch them to see if the chemo was working. This was His way of giving some sight to our faith.

Joe was scheduled for six one-week rounds of chemo with two weeks between each round. That meant the treatment would last almost five months, which seemed like a lifetime, but it helped me to think he would live at least five months to finish the treatment. I realize there was no logic to that thinking.

At the same time, we visited the radiologist about the high-beam guided radiation. This was a new machine that Lance Armstrong had raised funds to donate to a hospital that was just fifteen minutes away from us. At this time, there were only seven of these machines in the United States.

This doctor was one of the most encouraging doctors we have ever had. He believed it would work, even on Joe's pancreas—NO PROBLEM! He said he had used it on two other melanoma patients with great success. As regular radiation does not kill melanoma very well, he had our attention. We had seen the lack of results with regular radiation with Joe's dad. But this radiation could be set at an even higher intensity because it could be guided better.

At the time, our oncologist admitted he had not even heard about this type of radiation. He did not think we should do it because of the possibility of burning Joe's pancreas, where Joe had a large tumor that was unresponsive to the chemo, but we did it anyway. We felt God's Spirit had led us so we followed. Joe had only five treatments which each lasted only five minutes and it was gone!

Interestingly a year later, our oncologist moved into the same medical building right across the lobby from our radiologist. The oncologist said, "I thought you were crazy to get that radiation, but now I send everyone over there!" This was another reason I loved him so much. He gave us his opinion without making us feel compelled to follow it, and he was willing to learn. Perhaps he believed Joe was dying anyway, so he felt we could do whatever we thought was right. Whatever the case, we needed his kind of doctor.

31

**Mind Renewal**

**Lie:** God won't lead me contrary to everyone else's ideas, beliefs and solutions.

**Truth:** Psalm 23: *The Lord is MY Shepherd; He leads me and guides me.*

I can trust Him in me!

# Chapter 15

. . . . . . . . . . . . . . . . . . . . . . . . . . . . . . . . . . . . . . . . . . . . . . . . . . . . . . . . . . . . . . . .

## Resurrected Faith: Renewing the Promise

*If you abide in me and My words abide in you*
*ask whatever you wish and it will be done for you.*
*John 15:7*

Because we were basically shut-in, Joe and I watched a lot of faith preachers on television. If nothing else, they are people who believe that God can do anything. We were coming out of our little theological box of "cessationism," the belief that miraculous healings only occurred in Jesus' time to confirm His new revelation, and miracles ceased in that first generation of the church. It's funny how desperate need can give you a bigger God.

I started meeting with a dear friend and counselor at Operation 220, which is named after Galatians 2:20. I'm sure her ears were worn out. As much doubt, fear and confusion which could possibly be voiced in one hour was packed into each counseling session.

At one point she told me about her mom taking communion every morning so she could remember all that Jesus' blood bought for her. I grabbed on to this idea. So every morning I would sit and take grape juice and a cracker. "Christ in me" began to be bigger in my heart. I started to really embrace my union with Him. I was encouraged that before He died, Jesus' main prayer to His Father was for believers to see their oneness with Him and the Father. I also had access to His throne of grace because of His blood which speaks to the Father every day of my life.

John 17:11: *I am no longer in the world; and yet they themselves are in the world, and I come to You. Holy Father, keep them in Your name, the name which You have given Me, that they may be one even as We are.*

As I saw myself in Christ I started to feel more confident of the promise He gave me while Joe was in Pittsburgh.

*If you abide in Me and My words abide in you ask whatever you wish and it will be done for you.*

I was about to learn much more about the first part of the promise—the abiding part.

33

**Mind Renewal**

**Lie:** My faith makes things happen.

**Truth:** Ephesians 2:8: *For it is by grace you have been saved, through faith—and this not from yourselves, it is the gift of God—not by works, so that no one can boast.*

It's the work and grace of Christ that makes things happen!!

# Chapter 16

· · · · · · · · · · · · · · · · · · · · · · · · · · · · · · · · · · · · · · · · · · · · · · · · · · ·

# The Sting of the Cross

*But He was pierced through for our transgressions, He was crushed for our iniquities;*
*the chastening for our well-being fell upon Him, and by His scourging we are healed.*
*Isaiah 53:5*

As I started to abide in Christ and let Him abide in me, I started to receive from Him. I began laying my hands on Joe when I prayed. I laid my hands on the tumor lumps on his collar bone. We prayed out loud, "By His scourging we are healed," from Isaiah 53:5 and Matthew 8:17. I had always taken the gift of forgiveness of my sins and the gift of salvation. Nobody could talk me out of those gifts, but now I had added His healing gift from these "atonement" promises in Isaiah.

After one round of chemo on five consecutive days of treatment, the tumors on Joe's neck completely disappeared. Joe and I were so excited, but we did not tell anyone. My first thought was, "We need a PET scan."

The doctor said, "No, we usually do not do PET scans until the end of the six rounds of chemo." Perhaps he did not want me to be disappointed if I saw no change. Little did he know that I did not want him to give the credit to the chemo for what I knew God had done. So I insisted on the PET scan. He reluctantly agreed and Joe had the PET.

My desire was to show off God's power to the medical people. In the years since, several doctors have doubted that Joe ever had melanoma and insisted on seeing the actual pathology reports before they treated him. They found the story too amazing for a person to have Stage IV melanoma and live to tell about it.

---

### Mind Renewal

**Lie:** A miracle will guarantee others believe in Jesus—the doctors, and nurses who we love so much!

---

> **Truth:** Romans 1:20 & 25: *For since the creation of the world God's invisible qualities—his eternal power and divine nature—have been clearly seen, being understood from what has been made, so that men are without excuse. ... They exchanged the truth of God for a lie, and worshiped and served created things rather than the Creator—who is forever praised. Amen.*

We can see God's power and still not submit to Christ.

# Chapter 17

. . . . . . . . . . . . . . . . . . . . . . . . . . . . . . . . . . . . . . . . . . . . . . . . . . . . . . . .

## The Unbelievable Miracle

*So Peter was kept in the prison, but prayer for him was being made fervently by the church to God.*
*… When she recognized Peter's voice, because of her joy she did not open the gate, but ran in*
*and announced that Peter was standing in front of the gate. They said to her, "You are out of your*
*mind!" But she kept insisting that it was so. They kept saying, "It is his angel."*
*But Peter continued knocking; and when they had opened the door, they saw him and were amazed.*
*Acts 12:5, 15-16*

One practical thing we learned during this whole experience was to gather important medical records as soon as possible and carry them with us. That helped us connect with new doctors immediately and we were spared many days of waiting. So we made sure to get the pictures from this latest PET scan. We even had them before our oncologist. Joe and I couldn't resist looking at them under our kitchen light, as if we could actually read a scan. Soon I was in tears. All my hopes were gone. The cancer was totally out of control, as there were dark spots all over Joe's body.

The next day when I saw the oncologist in the hall, he could tell I was upset and asked what was wrong. I told him the cancer had spread. He wondered how I knew. I told him we had looked at the images from the PET scan. He gave me a funny look and said, "Let's go look at it together." We went into Joe's chemo room and placed the pictures under the x-ray lights. I proceeded to show him the spots where I saw cancer. He laughed and said, "Well, that one is his heart." Then he continued looking and said, "But there is some here … and more here … and here."

At that exact moment his nurse walked in. She was telling us that we should read the report sent by the actual radiologist! Both the doctor and I kept looking at the scans and ignoring her. She finally yelled at us that the report says, "NED—No evidence of disease!" It was a clear scan—Joe was cancer free. We both turned to look at her. The doctor left the room with the report, and Joe and I cried knowing "God's chemo" had worked! The doctor walked back in and said, "We need to leave the reading of scans to the radiologist." Humble pie was being served to all of us—and we all gladly ate it.

The first person I thought of was Rhoda in Acts 12 trying to tell the disciples that Peter had just been delivered from jail and was knocking at the door and their prayers had been immediately answered. They didn't believe her. That nurse was our Rhoda.

As you can tell by now, our faith was mixed with a lot of doubt. Still, God carried us through. We were so excited, to the point of stopping treatment. The nurses came in the room and tried to set up the next chemo appointment. I was sort of struggling with them anyway, and it all came out at that moment. I told them that they did not give me any hope. Later, two of them came back into the room and apologized but said they had worked in oncology for 10 years and had never seen an advanced melanoma patient respond to this treatment. They did not want to raise my hopes. I forgave them because I realized the treatment was their best human hope. God was our hope. We decided to finish the treatment, believing God was using it. We were excited and others shared the excitement with us but we could tell most people, especially the doctor, believed the cancer was going to return. From the human's standpoint, Joe was still not out of the woods.

## Mind Renewal

**Lie:** God needs my faith to MAKE Him real and for Him to answer prayer.

**Truth:** 2 Timothy 2:11-13: *It is a trustworthy statement: For if we died with Him, we will also live with Him; If we endure, we will also reign with Him; If we deny Him, He also will deny us; If we are faithless, He remains faithful, for He cannot deny Himself.*

## Chapter 18

. . . . . . . . . . . . . . . . . . . . . . . . . . . . . . . . . . . . . . . . . . . . . . . . . . . . .

# His Saints, My Delight

*As for the saints who are in the earth, they are the majestic ones in whom is all my delight.*
*Psalm 16:3*

Being a pastor's wife was an experience that could fill a book of its own.
Before all this happened, I had been wondering what church should look
like. I had written this in my devotional time a year before.

> How committed am I to **Your** church,
> **Your** body on earth?
> Is it just an organization,
> a club full of people, "fellowshipping?"
> Or is it . . .
> **Your** Body imprinted with nail holes,
> crowned with thorns,
> reaching out with resurrected life,
> *emptied* of self-gratification,
> self-indulgence, self-interest, self-protection . . .
> *filled* with **Your** heart beating through us,
> touching each other's brokenness,
> letting **Your** healing restore us
> as we open the Church's doors
> to each other more and more?

I was one of those people who had high hopes for the church. Yet I had put
a standard on it that was way above the one Christ had placed on it. I didn't
know it would be painful. I thought everyone would be truthful and loving
and never say the wrong thing, including me. Grace would be the air we
breathe and everyone would agree on what the Bible says. Where all this came
from I do not know. The minute I enter any church, that particular church has
a much greater potential of being hurt by my imperfection.

I remember calling a friend who felt more like a sister, who had left our
church a year before. She had not yet called me about Joe, but I knew she was

genuinely concerned about our family. She mistakenly believed that I would not want her to call because she had left our church. I was hurt when she didn't call. I finally picked up the phone and called her (and yelled at her for not calling). She had always given me the "okay" to disagree with her without fearing rejection. And she always brought out feistiness in me, but truth was—I needed her.

To me the church is God's people—not the building or the group you worship with. What I need for fellowship is truthfulness in relationships and this sister always gave that to me. Truthfulness opens doors for real fellowship with Jesus between me and my sisters. I am learning that even worshipping in the same building does not necessarily mean we have been fellowshipping with each other. Jesus said that He desires true worshippers who worship in Spirit and in truth. Friendships around Jesus built on Spirit and truth are a real gift. We can disagree and even argue over belief systems and feel safe. He's our glue.

### Mind Renewal

**Lie:** The Church must be perfect in order for God to work through it!

**Truth:** Philippians 4:2: *I plead with Euodia and I plead with Syntyche to agree with each other in the Lord. Yes, and I ask you, loyal yokefellow, help these women who have contended at my side in the cause of the gospel, along with Clement and the rest of my fellow workers, whose names are in the book of life.*

The church has always been messy and filled with disagreements and struggles, but we can get through them.

# Chapter 19

. . . . . . . . . . . . . . . . . . . . . . . . . . . . . . . . . . . . . . . . . . . . . . . . . . . . . . . . . . . . . . .

## My Burden Bearers

*For my yoke is easy and my burden is light.*
*Matthew 11:30*

I had many close friends who have the "gift of faith." God always seems to give me a person with this gift when He walks me through a difficult time. Friends with this gift helped me believe Joe was not going to die. Their faith did not come from mere wishful thinking. It was solid, by God's Spirit, strong and sure.

One friend had the gift of faith to the point of exhorting Joe to keep living when he said he wanted to stop all treatments and began preparing his funeral. She said simply, "Your kids need you, your wife needs you, and your church needs you." She was herself and Jesus came through her in a big way because she shared her heart. We believe this was a turning point for Joe to fight to want to live while in such pain. The Lord broke through and Joe "found" and started to quote this passage:

Philippians 2:20-26: *Now as always Christ will be exalted in my body, whether by life or by death. For to me, to live is Christ and to die is gain. If I am to go on living in the body, this will mean fruitful labor for me. Yet what shall I choose? I do not know! I am torn between the two: I desire to depart and be with Christ, which is better by far; but it is more necessary for you that I remain in the body. Convinced of this, I know that I will remain, and I will continue with all of you for your progress and joy in the faith, so that through my being with you again your joy in Christ Jesus will overflow on account of me.*

These words were LIFE because God was leading them at that time for us. They were not magical and a formula for healing. I look now at Stronghold Ministry and can see that Joe has given Christ's Good News to so many that are going through the same. Many cancer patients needed him too! (Hindsight is so fun!)

Another dear friend (the one who arranged for the free trip to Costa Rica) helped in so many ways. She was always available to watch the kids. Sometimes she stayed in the hospital with Joe as his night nurse. I was sometimes afraid

41

she was taking on too much, so I tried to only ask for what I needed most—night nursing and kid watching. I had nothing to give her at the time and I didn't want her to become burned out. Looking back, I realize she took on more than I knew as people often called her for details, not wanting to "bother" me. I so love her heart and trust God has and will reward her for her faithfulness when His Spirit led her to serve our family.

I would have welcomed the calls of anyone who was interested in the details we were going through, because my "love language" is words. Knowing a person's love language really is a plus when trying to help. I am sometimes bad at this though. I tend to give out of my own love language. I am a talker and a listener. The phone is my love language. Cards and flowers did not speak as loudly to my heart as a short conversation centered on hope and faith. (Don't get me wrong, I really appreciated the cards and goodies!) I loved those short phone calls when I just cried and shared my doubts and was encouraged that Joe was not going to die.

I still value daily calls from sisters who just share their struggles or victories with me. It's the daily walking with Jesus while cooking or in traffic. I have a few friends who live miles away who still give me those calls. This keeps me centered on Jesus during storms. My daughter, Amy, sees Jesus in the simplest things and often calls to tell me how she has seen Him. I have grown to love cell phones because they give me the opportunity to hear from Him through my Christian family.

I realize a lot of men give their wives the job of caring and finding out the details of sick people. God chooses friends, supporters and comforters for our needs and it might be different than we expect. Yet God Himself is our ultimate comforter and "the God of all comfort." Any comfort we get is from His hand.

I could name many more loving sisters that gave to me. In fact, I was often overwhelmed by His love that came through His burden bearers.

### Mind Renewal

**Lie:** God's comfort must come in the ways I prefer.

**Truth:** Colossians 4:8: *For I have sent him to you for this very purpose, that you may know about our circumstances and that he may encourage your hearts.*

# Chapter 20

. . . . . . . . . . . . . . . . . . . . . . . . . . . . . . . . . . . . . . . . . . . . . . . . . . . . . . . . . . . . . .

## Basketball—Not So Bad After All

*Indeed, the LORD will comfort Zion; He will comfort all her waste places.*
*Isaiah 51:3*

I have learned lots about the male species through all of this. Before cancer, I felt like sports were pulling my family apart even when we were in the same building doing sports. I judged Joe every time he went to play basketball. Because Joe loves basketball so much our kids were on the school basketball teams as well as in community basketball leagues. I felt like we had spent most of our lives in a gym. Joe also played basketball himself twice a week. Many times I had told him this seemed so unbalanced. "You always come home hurt. Where's the fun in that?" He would just look at me like I was not really living life.

In my mind, basketball was redeemed by the Lord through the cancer. Joe's basketball friends emailed Joe daily and came to see him often. One of the guy's daughters was diagnosed with cancer at the same time. They encouraged each other a lot.

One of the guys had lost his wife to breast cancer after an 11-year battle. He is one who told us to look for those who pray boldly and believe strongly in healing. In his experience, the elders in his church did not pray in faith for his wife. He said they prayed for encouragement, patience and all the great Christian virtues needed to get through trials, but they would not pray for healing. He came to Joe's bed and prayed for healing loud and clear. God used this man to lift me up.

I have grown to love basketball and watching football. I am learning that there is an unseen bonding during those games among men. Not many words shared, but when they are, it is with loud voices, joking and kidding. In the end, however, big hugs speak loudly when the real trials come upon their team.

**Mind Renewal**

**Lie:** Things which I do not value are not valuable for God's purposes. So it is right to judge "stuff."

**Truth:** 1 Corinthian 4:5: *Therefore, judge nothing before the appointed time; wait till the Lord comes. He will bring to light what is hidden in darkness and will expose the motives of men's hearts. At that time each will receive his praise from God.*

I mistakenly tend to declare "neutral, everyday life" as either good or bad, spiritual or not.

# Chapter 21

......................................................

## Walking Together by Faith, Hope and Love

*But eagerly desire the greater gifts.*
*And now I will show you the most excellent way.*
1 Corinthians 12:31

I had little patience with those who were "hoping" for a miracle. I wanted to be around those who *believed* in a miracle. I was the church's biggest critic. I did not have that warm fuzzy type of love that hugs or that soft humming voice that makes people feel all gooey. And in the flesh, I can be mistrusting, cynical and full of judgments.

Yet a weird thing happened with the anger and frustration I had during this time. I felt Jesus holding me harder and loving me deeper and I saw this in the Christians around me as well. They let me vent. They let me cry. They let me not give to them. They let me doubt. They let me suffer and struggle without judgment. (If they *were* judging me, they hid it well).

Cancer woke me up to Christ's words when He said that He came for the sick and the sinner, not those who had it all together. Joe and I were the sick and the sinner and most Christians do not want their pastors to be the sick and sinner. My niece seemed to get this picture. She had been in a church whose pastor admitted he was having homosexual affairs and another leader had a different problem. She noted that when leaders fall they lose their jobs, their church, their friends—everything. However, when a sheep falls, all the church reaches out to help. They even try to restore the sheep. I looked at her and felt Jesus' love.

Some of the ways I saw our church reach out to us were through individuals that let me be myself. I remember telling one brother, "Please quit praying 'God's will be done.'" I wanted him to pray for God to completely heal Joe. This wise, older man simply changed his prayer in my presence. He did not argue theology with me.

Another brother passed me one day as I was venting fear. He said, "God doesn't give no snakes." (He has since told me that he said *stones*, but I heard *snakes* probably because I felt that snake, Satan, breathing down my neck).

45

Those simple words helped me stand again on the promise of healing which God had given me.

Luke 11:11: *Now suppose one of you fathers is asked by his son for a fish; he will not give him a snake instead of a fish, will he?*

Matthew 7:9: *Or what man is there among you who, when his son asks for a loaf, will give him a stone?*

God's Word timely spoken kept me fighting the good fight of faith. Christians I barely knew sent me Bible verses in the mail, allowing me to see the larger body of Christ in action. One family sent a card once a month just to remind us of their prayers. I was never around this family at that time, yet I posted each promise they claimed for us on my kitchen cupboard. Many others sent dinners, maids, money, plane tickets, and phone calls. God was reaching out to me through His church with a grace I had never experienced before. These were His saints in the spiritual battle with us.

Our little church had faithful elders who stayed with us through a hard time for our church. God used them greatly. They could have been in a more exciting church, but chose to stick it out in a church where the pastor needed help. Hopefully, they did not feel trapped. I pray God blesses each one who walked with us and Him during this time. I know what was given through Christ will not burn and they will be rewarded.

James 5:4: *Is anyone among you sick? Then he must call for the elders of the church and they are to pray over him, anointing him with oil in the name of the Lord; and the prayer offered in faith will restore the one who is sick, and the Lord will raise him up, and if he has committed sins, they will be forgiven him.*

They applied their shaky faith every time they prayed. We all applied our shaky faith every time we prayed. I believe their obedience to this prayer and healing ministry given to elders of the church was instrumental to Joe's healing. Since Joe's healing, many people have come to us for prayer after going to their own churches whose leadership does not practice this part of Scripture. It's a great verse to read, but standing on it can put a person in the battle.

This is one part of the amazing inheritance given to his children in Christ. It's one of those gifts we should really desire to open.

I am eternally thankful for those in our little church who walked so intimately with us!

**Mind Renewal**

**Lie:** A pastor should not be a burden on the church he serves.

**Truth:** Matthew 25:36, 40: I was sick, and you visited Me. ... Truly I say to you, to the extent that you did it to one of these brothers of Mine, *even the least of them*, you did it to Me.

# Part 2

············································································

## Lessons Learned

### Gems I have learned about abiding in Him.

*If you abide in Me, and My words abide in you,*
*ask whatever you wish, and it will be done for you.*
*John 15:7*

# Chapter 22

. . . . . . . . . . . . . . . . . . . . . . . . . . . . . . . . . . . . . . . . . . . . . . . . . . . . . . . . . . . . . . . . . . .

## Abiding Secrets I Have Learned

*Peace I leave with you; My peace I give to you; not as the world gives do I give to you.*
*Do not let your heart be troubled, nor let it be fearful.*
*John 14:27*

By Christmas 2008, the five year anniversary of finding the melanoma, we had three scares of its return. Cancer never really has an ending in one's life. It's the first thought when any health problem arises. One day I told someone that Joe had pain in his stomach for quite a while. Their immediate question was, "Do you think the cancer is back?"

We have been thankful Joe is alive, but we also realized that the chemo and radiation took a toll on his body. He has had five additional surgeries for scar tissue and other complications. He has thrown his back out playing basketball, and he had to deal with the addictive qualities of pain medicine and its other side effects. He is dealing with a weaker body and pain which doctors told him may be due to the cancer, chemo and radiation. We have more pictures of the inside of his body than the outside.

The hardest part though was sometimes when he shared about his pain he felt he was a burden to others, or even judged for hurting so often. So cancer has had a lasting sting even though there is a great outcome. Yet Jesus says our weakness is our strength because He lives well through a vessel of weakness. Paul actually says to boast in our weakness:

2 Corinthians 12:9: *And He has said to me, "My grace is sufficient for you, for power is perfected in weakness." Most gladly, therefore, I will rather boast about my weaknesses, so that the power of Christ may dwell in me.*

A friend shared that she had a dream early on that Joe was going to be healed but that his body was going to be his thorn. The beauty of this thought is that Joe will probably attract people who need and embrace this truth about weakness.

We are walking lightly on this ground we call life. We are all going to die. Cancer reminds us that someday death is going to take our earthly lives. Cancer forces us to face reality. I have begun to define life a little differently than breathing and a heartbeat.

John 5:24: *Truly, truly, I say to you, he who hears My word, and believes Him who sent Me, has eternal life, and does not come into judgment, but has passed out of death into life.*

According to this verse, if I believe in Jesus, I am already walking in eternal life. I wonder if passing into the next life is like continuing to walk with Jesus in the full light of who He is.

John 3:15: *Whoever believes will in Him have eternal life.*

Life is in His Son, Jesus Christ. He *is* eternal Life. We have it now in Him. Sometimes those words seem academic or just theology—not real. It's funny how God draws us to real life so we know Jesus more deeply. As I draw on His Spirit in me, something comes to life in me. I can walk with a peace which only He can give.

*Chapter 23*

. . . . . . . . . . . . . . . . . . . . . . . . . . . . . . . . . . . . . . . . . . . . . . . . . . . . . . . . .

# Abiding Faith

*For as many as are the promises of God, in Him they are yes;*
*therefore also through Him is our Amen to the glory of God through us.*
*2 Corinthians 1:20*

Time passes. Years go by and Joe is alive—we are alive. I do not take that for granted anymore. Why Joe was healed and another person isn't is something I cannot explain. I've watched some amazing people pass—people we prayed for many times *in faith.*

Still, I do know I am no longer shy to ask boldly for healing for those who come to us with cancer. We stand in prayer for each person until the end—whether healed on earth or in heaven.

Yet a huge part of the promise He gave me was learning the meaning of "abiding in Him." The ministry all people need is encouragement to ABIDE IN CHRIST. That is where His life is. This is where God's promises abide.

Abiding is a moment-by-moment experience—in the *present* moment. When I look at the past, I can think of lots that I didn't do or say right. When I look at the future, sometimes fears overtake me. I realize the longer I walk the Christian life, the way gets narrower. Jesus says He is the way, the truth and the life. I need to draw from His power and life moment by moment, fixing my eyes on Him, the Author and Finisher of my faith. The more I get to know His voice and His heart the more I experience eternal life on this side. He is becoming my refuge and my stronghold on this side of eternity. The more I see Him the more death loses its sting.

Abiding in Christ means recklessly following Him wherever He leads, being aware of His presence and love for me all day long. It is abandonment to Him, knowing He is good and He is powerful. And He is my friend.

Following Him makes me laugh a little. Think about this: He was born in a barn; touched a person with leprosy; "rearranged the furniture" at the church; got wildly excited over a widow's almost worthless coin given to His Father; made friends with a person in a tree; and he let a woman wash and then dry his feet ... with her hair. His path can go in strange places with strange causes and stranger results. He's a little weird and He loves the weird.

Yet I seem to want Him to lead me to the comfortable or "happening" place (not the weird one). The place where there is no pain, no suffering, no struggle. The popular places of this world: successful jobs, successful children, successful friends, the places where everyone wants to be. There, I can easily follow.

I have a harder time abandoning myself to Him in places of less comfort and where I am out of control. Places with little praise and few stars for my behavior chart; places where the sick and weak have names and faces. Places where I have to let Him love through me because my own love falls short. I do not want to walk where I do not look like a winner. But when I fight surrendering to Jesus, I lose the chance to see His life in action.

For now, for today, He has granted for Joe to live and not die. He led others to leave this earth and go live with Him face-to-face. Surrender looks different for everyone. His voice leads each of us on different paths. I can't always understand why, but I do know I need to abide in His love and only then can I lead others to truth without worrying about their outcomes.

I resolve to walk with Him and abide in His love in all the places He calls me.

# Chapter 24

. . . . . . . . . . . . . . . . . . . . . . . . . . . . . . . . . . . . . . . . . . . . . . . . . . . . . . . . . . . . . . . . . . . . . . .

## Abiding in His Voice

*You can do nothing without Me*
*John 15:5*

I don't do well with conditions. If it is up to me to do ANYTHING, I usually fail. I have proven Jesus' words over and over, "You can do nothing without Me" (John 15:5). Left to myself, I have no love for anyone. I am self-protective and self-caring. I wanted Joe to live for a lot of selfish reasons. He takes care of me. I can talk to him. He gives me some identity (Joe's wife). I wanted him to raise the kids and pay for their college. Financially, I feel secure with his ability to provide. It's ugly when I see how little I believe God will take care of me and fulfill my life apart from Joe. So how can I believe He will hear my cry?

My true concept of God was revealed through Joe's cancer. I was often driven by fear, guilt and making deals with God. Old voices urged me to do all the right things to make God move. When I'm not trusting God and living out of my own schemes, what the Bible calls "walking in the flesh," I can be very manipulative. My relationship with God had been based on my own goodness and ability to live out certain Christian rules. My performance was the focus. I made things happen. I knew "Jesus" was the answer to every question, but I did not let Him be my life, to live out from me. This is what my religion looked like: read the Bible and then obey it. The silly thing is that I never could really do what it said because my attitudes would show.

His promise to me had a condition I had not understood before: ABIDING IN Him. The cancer battle helped me learn how to let Him live in me, and I in Him on a daily, hourly, and moment-by-moment basis.

I read about Saul who was the king the people wanted instead of God. Saul always tried to be one step ahead of God. Samuel the prophet would give Saul directions from God and Saul would add to those directions. He always wanted to do more or different than what God clearly asked. One example was when Saul was told to fight a battle in a certain way:

1 Samuel 15:3: *Now go and strike Amalek and utterly destroy all that he has, and do not spare him; but put to death both man and woman, child and infant, ox and sheep, camel and donkey.*

But Saul decided to go with his own exceptions:

1 Samuel 15:6: *Saul said to the Kenites, "Go, depart, go down from among the Amalekites, so that I do not destroy you with them; for you showed kindness to all the sons of Israel when they came up from Egypt." So the Kenites departed from among the Amalekites.*

Saul preferred to save these people because they had been good to him. But God did not tell him so.

At another time Saul took the animals from the spoils of a battle and offered them to God as a sacrifice. All this sounds holy and right. But God ended up telling him,

Samuel 15:22-23: *Has the LORD as much delight in burnt offerings and sacrifices as in obeying the voice of the LORD? Behold, to obey is better than sacrifice, and to heed than the fat of rams. ... For rebellion is as the sin of divination, and insubordination is as iniquity and idolatry. Because you have rejected the word of the LORD, He has also rejected you from being king.*

In my opinion, I don't think Saul even saw himself as being rebellious. He probably thought he was pleasing God by going the extra mile.

As I meditate on Saul's mistake, I see me. I think I can offer God some good thing, an even better thing, to show my love. What He really wants is for me to take HIS GOOD THING and let that be enough.

**His good thing is Jesus Christ!**

I am learning to unwrap this gift of Him daily.

*Chapter 25*

. . . . . . . . . . . . . . . . . . . . . . . . . . . . . . . . . . . . . . . . . . . . . . . . . . . . . . . . . . . .

# Abiding in His Finished Work

*Therefore when Jesus had received the sour wine, He said, "It is finished!"*
*And He bowed His head and gave up His spirit.*
*John 19:30*

If you have ever had a hard deadline for a project to be finished, you know how it feels when that date has come and gone. You can't go back. You can't add to it or change it. You either made the deadline or you missed it.

I think that is what Jesus was saying on the cross after He received the sour wine for pain. He took the last sip of human compassion and realized it could not fix His situation. It could not change His situation and it did not have the power to deliver. He then said "It is Finished," and gave up His spirit. He was totally in the hands and purpose of His Father, the God of the Universe.

At that point creation, history, and life came to rest. Jesus was doing the work no human could do: redemption.

- He paid the price to bring us to God.
- He emptied Himself to fill us with His Spirit.
- He became what God would use to release His inheritance into this world to His saints.
- He did what we never could do.

And He said, "It is finished!"

Now as a believer, I am given a major work—the work of becoming a RECEIVER of His finished work on that cross.

My main job as a believer is to unwrap what God gave me that day when Jesus said, "It is finished."

I am not to add to that work ...

all my good deeds,
right devotion,
right theology,
any "math" that says,
Jesus plus this or that = God's love and favor.

This is a battle of faith, not works.

John 6:28: *Therefore they said to Him, "What shall we do, so that we may work the works of God?" Jesus answered and said to them, "This is the work of God that you believe in Him whom He has sent."*

I have had to wake up each day (during the cancer and ever since) and ask myself if I agree with Jesus when He said, "It is finished." Is His work enough for me? Do I walk this day *beside* Him, making my own way, looking for my own comfort, trying to gain a righteousness that gains me points? Or do I agree with Him and walk IN HIS FINISHED WORK?

- Agreeing with all He says I have in Him—forgiveness, acceptance, approval, healing, peace, joy, patience, etc.
- Agreeing with who He says I am.
- Agreeing to know He is the only Life that pleased The Father completely and yet has been given freely to me.

On one hand, it all seems so simple, because it is.

I have found the battle is always at the foot of the cross—receiving that work or rejecting that work. Am I trying to get the teacher to extend the due date on the work that needs to be done? He won't extend it. He will only present the finished project to me for my grade and it's always an A. It's His A. I can take that A, or try again. But why would I do that?

Hebrews 4:11: *Let us labor therefore to enter into that rest, lest any man fall after the same example of unbelief.*

# Chapter 26

. . . . . . . . . . . . . . . . . . . . . . . . . . . . . . . . . . . . . . . . . . . . . . . . . . . . . . . . . . . . . . . . . . . .

## Abiding in His Ownership of Me

*For He rescued me from the domain of darkness,*
*and transferred me to the kingdom of His beloved Son.*
*Colossians 1:13*

Raised Catholic, I learned a lot of things about Jesus that are right, but I also learned (or heard in my weird way) a lot of things that were wrong. One belief I picked up was that I needed to confess my sins before I died or I would go to hell. I also believed that I had to go to confession with a priest or it wouldn't count as true confession. I tried to sin very little and then to keep up by confessing those sins I did commit. Yet around age 16 it hit me that I was never going to be good enough. I gave up trying and just felt bad about myself every day.

When I was 17, a friend shared that I could place my trust in Jesus as my Savior, ask Him into my heart, and He would forgive me forever and then I would definitely go to heaven. I remember arguing with her, "So I could do that just one time and that would be enough to go to heaven?" She said yes. "So I could sin right after that and still go to heaven?" Yes.

I laughed at her and told her I did not believe that. But as I walked away from her I thought, "I would be stupid not to ask Him to live in me if that is all it takes." So I did. I asked Him into my heart. I remember immediately feeling so light. I can still go to that place. A load was taken away. A love came upon me which made me feel for the first time that I did not need anyone else's approval —not even my own! The feeling lasted for a while, but the assurance has lasted my whole life. I believe that Jesus did come into my very scattered, dark heart that day and changed it and He has never left. It was not a great show. In fact, nobody knew I did that for years. It was His seed of life. I had no mentoring or "discipleship," no one to tell me what to do next. I did not even own a Bible, but that day I experienced His presence and believed I was loved and okay. I forever belonged to Him and heaven.

Facing death with Joe brought back those old questions, "Can I know for sure I'm going to heaven? Have I believed in vain?" Yet I experienced that same

Presence during this trial of cancer. I am His, so I can rest. Abiding in His ownership brings peace when I am having an anxiety attack (and I have many). Now I say, "Lord, this anxious child of yours is scared and fearful." I hear Him whisper, "But you are *My* anxious child and even now your anxiety (though it is full of disbelief and sin and everything false) will not separate you from My love."

- No condemnation from Him.
- No judgment from Him.
- No separation from Him.
- No hiding from Him.

I was put into His kingdom that day and I cannot be booted out. He gave me the Kingdom of His beloved Son and I am learning to live there with and *in Him* today.

# Chapter 27

. . . . . . . . . . . . . . . . . . . . . . . . . . . . . . . . . . . . . . . . . . . . . . . . . . . . . .

## Abiding in His Gift of Prayer

*Therefore let us draw near with confidence to the throne of grace,*
*so that we may receive mercy and find grace to help in time of need.*
Hebrews 4:16

Prayer is one of those funny Christian disciplines. I used it a lot when Joe was in the heat of the battle. I was often tempted to use it for righteousness and to try to win God's ears. I am sure this came from how I was raised in religion. I remember saying certain prayers over and over when I would get in trouble. I guess that was a way of hoping He would hear me. It was almost like chanting. Jesus told His disciples many words would not make a difference when talking to Him; neither would repeating the same words.

He was kind enough to bring me to desperation so I would just cry out for mercy and grace.

Now, before I pray I try to make a conscious decision to RECEIVE Christ's work on the cross. I have to decide I can approach God boldly because of Christ's finished work. I sometimes believe there are a ton of conditions for being heard. Yet there is something about standing IN Christ that meets any condition.

- I am not looking to my own righteousness to be heard.
- I am not cleaning up my life to approach God.
- My prayers are not manipulations to move God.
- I do not have to say prayers in a certain way.

Philippians 3:9: *Not having a righteousness of my own derived from the Law, but that which is through faith in Christ, the righteousness which comes from God on the basis of faith.*

Romans 13:14: *Put on the Lord Jesus Christ, and make no provision for the flesh in regard to its lusts.*

This verse helps me see that as I approach God I need to "put on" all that was freely given me in Jesus. I need not approach God with my own clothes of

61

"rightness" or goodness. God sees me dressed in what He has provided for me to live in—the life of His Son. The boldness and freedom in these clothes are beautiful and fit perfectly. I am noticed and heard by the One whose attention is most important.

Here again I had to let go of my religious lessons on prayer. Beliefs like: first I need to repent, then be thankful, then search my motives, and only then ask. This would be the formula that would somehow guarantee I was heard. But I am heard because of the formula God made with His secret ingredient—His Son. I have Him all day long. At any moment I need Him or just want to enjoy Him, He's there.

Prayer is no longer me "going" to Him. Rather it's me acknowledging that He has come near to me, walking with me and sharing hearts with each other.

# Chapter 28

.........................................................................

## Abiding in His Guilt Offering for Me

*Who is the one who condemns? Christ Jesus is He who died, yes, rather who was raised,*
*who is at the right hand of God, who also intercedes for us.*
*Romans 8:34*

One of the greatest fights I had during and after the cancer is with "false guilt." I grew up guilty. Mainly, I was guilty of being not perfect. When I have a problem in any relationship it is usually because I did not meet an expectation, either my own, theirs or God's. To always feel guilty and never feel okay is false guilt. I have a few choices of how to handle this:

1. Blame others and God for too high expectations.
2. Self-condemn and try to change.
3. Let someone else defend me and fight for me.

I'm going with the third choice. I am learning to receive the testimony about myself from Jesus. One of His gifts is that He is now seated next to God making intercession for me.

I can picture this dialogue in heaven. I can imagine Him looking straight in the Father's face and smiling at the lies. "I paid for her, she is ours, and she's okay. She has My Gift of Righteousness all over her."

Romans 8:34: *Who is the one who condemns? Christ Jesus is He who died, yes, rather who was raised, who is at the right hand of God, who also intercedes for us.*

And ...

Hebrews 10:12: *But He, having offered one sacrifice for sins for all time, sat down at the right hand of God.*

And ...

Revelation 12:10: *Then I heard a loud voice in heaven, saying, "Now the salvation, and the power, and the kingdom of our God and the authority of His Christ have come, for the accuser of our brethren has been thrown down, he who accuses them before our God day and night."*

This verse has become a major comfort. My freedom from guilt was announced in a LOUD VOICE ... IN HEAVEN. It's true! I am learning to let Jesus fight these accusations and not even try to approach them on a reasoning basis.

## Chapter 29

· · · · · · · · · · · · · · · · · · · · · · · · · · · · · · · · · · · · · · · · · · · · · · · · · · · · · ·

## Abiding in His Authority in My Battles

*This day the Lord will deliver you up into my hands, and I will strike you down and remove your head from you. And I will give the dead bodies of the army of the Philistines this day to the birds of the sky and the wild beasts of the earth, that all the earth may know that there is a God in Israel, and that all this assembly may know that the Lord does not deliver by sword or by spear; for the battle is the Lord's and He will give you into our hands.*

1 Samuel 17:46

Receiving Christ's authority is one of those works. I do not make Him have authority. He already has it. I do not need to yell in a loud voice to fight my enemy. He is already speaking to the Father for me moment-by-moment.

Ephesians 1:20: *He raised Him from the dead and seated Him at His right hand in the heavenly places.*

And…

Ephesians 2:6: *He raised **us** up with Him, and seated **us** with Him in the heavenly places in Christ Jesus.*

And…

Colossians 3:1: *Therefore if you have been raised up with Christ, keep seeking the things above, where Christ is, seated at the right hand of God.*

I am seated in a different place now. I need to *stay seated* and not strive when fighting battles. This is an eternal resting spot which started when I first believed in Him.

I am also learning to "stand" from Ephesians 6:13. Neither sitting nor standing require movement, but being anchored in what Jesus has done for us.

Ephesians 6:13: *Therefore put on the full armor of God, so that when the day of evil comes, you may be able to stand your ground, and after you have done everything, to stand.*

Stand firm.

# Chapter 30

......................................................................................

## Abiding in Jesus as Friend

*No longer do I call you slaves, for the slave does not know what his master is doing; but I have called*
*you friends, for all things that I have heard from My Father I have made known to you.*
*John 15:15*

One of the greatest lessons I learned in the cancer trial was that God actually wanted to lead me day by day. He was and is my friend. I had been relating to Him more as a master than a friend. It was more of a fearful relationship than one of caring and love, and full of religion. I would do things for Him because He was God and I should, rather than because He was safe and leading me. I was always *trying* to be obedient.

I do not know what He wants for others. I only know how He leads me each day. This is why I cannot say everyone will be healed. I can say that everyone can have HIS friendship and He will lead them to the treatments and doctors He wants for them. I have come to realize each person has his or her own relationship with Him. And the same is true for that person's family. My strong desire is to encourage all to hear from Him. I always ask, "Has He spoken to you about what promises He wants to give you?"

Though I do not know where He is leading others, I *do* know His cross is where His gifts begin and end. As children we can go to Him and unwrap them as He gives them to us specifically. He desires to make known to us all that He has heard from His Father. Our part is to listen and believe He wants to speak to us as friends.

Ultimately, He is the one who opens ears to hear. We can learn a lot about Him, but He has to open ears. I believe He opens mine every day as I desire to know Him. When my ears are dull with the worries of this world, I need to take time to still the voices and noise, opening the eyes of my heart more than the eyes of my mind.

Isaiah 50:4: *He awakens Me morning by morning, He awakens My ear to listen as a disciple. The Lord GOD has opened My ear; And I was not disobedient nor did I turn.*

There were so many days I saw Him lead us. He used a stranger on a day we were helplessly lost in a huge hospital and Joe could barely walk. A woman found us a wheelchair and took us right to the place in the hospital where we needed to be. She came out of nowhere and then disappeared. People said to us, "How did you get that wheelchair? We have been waiting for one for 30 minutes." I started to see Him in the smallest things. He was and is our Good Shepherd and Friend. He takes our hand and walks us in paths we don't even know exist.

John 10:27: *My sheep hear My voice, and I know them, and they follow Me.*

## Chapter 31

......................................................................................................

## Abiding in His Approval

*Listen to Me, you who know righteousness, a people in whose heart is My law;*
*Do not fear the reproach of man, nor be dismayed at their reviling.*
Isaiah 51:7

One of the biggest stumbling blocks in my life is wanting people's approval. I still deal with this every day. I was a pastor's wife, and from the outside, that might look like a great place to be. I have found it to be the opposite.

Sometimes I became like a person's mom (in their mind). Now, we all love our moms, but we surely do not want to be mothered when we are grown and on our own. Moms are sometimes not treated with a lot of approval. We love them, but we want some separation (unless they can meet needs for us). So I dealt with people trying to level the ground when I was just giving an opinion—just like they were giving theirs. Sometimes people would make me "bad" so that they could disagree with me. Some wanted everyone else to know how bad I was and how strong I am to disagree with. I had a choice. I could take the false identity given to me and to try to become invisible to make people happy. Or I could hide behind what Jesus says about me and let the approval of man be left to them.

Now by no means do I think I was perfect with everyone. I had moments of anger and offensiveness with people. Yet even when I am wrong, I still need to lean on the approval of God.

There are many other places this shows up in my life:

- Being a parent.
- Being a wife.
- Being a friend.
- Being a Christian.

I am growing in the area of not fearing the reproach of man, nor being dismayed at their reviling.

During the cancer I felt people's love and care. They were willing to give me grace. I did not have to be perfect. They felt sorry for me. We were the underdog. It was strange.

68

I felt it was easier to gain people's approval when Joe had cancer. Maybe this is why Jesus had to ask the man by the healing pool if he truly wanted to get well. You might be treated differently… if you're not sick.

During the cancer, my greatest fight for man's approval was over my theology of healing. I had to fight through different theological views to receive Christ's healing for Joe. I finally gave up the fight in my head and started to cling to the things He specifically showed me.

He held on to me when I was weak at believing. It was His gift to give, and I did not have to earn it. I could again rest in His finished work—not my faith or right theology according to the opinion of others.

Letting go of people's approval and living in God's approval is a gift He is giving me each day. I am learning to suffer the loss of my reputation, friendships and understanding, because I already have HIS approval.

Think of how Jesus had to fight this same battle with the approval of man. I meditate on Isaiah 50 whenever I am having a pity party about being mistreated or misunderstood.

Isaiah 50:6-10: *I gave My back to those who strike Me, and My cheeks to those who pluck out the beard; I did not cover My face from humiliation and spitting. For the Lord GOD helps Me, Therefore, I am not disgraced; Therefore, I have set My face like flint, and I know that I will not be ashamed. He who vindicates Me is near; who will contend with Me? Let us stand up to each other; who has a case against Me? Let him draw near to Me. Behold, the Lord GOD helps Me; Who is he who condemns Me? Behold, they will all wear out like a garment; The moth will eat them. Who is among you that fears the LORD, that obeys the voice of His servant, that walks in darkness and has no light? Let him trust in the name of the LORD and rely on his God.*

# Chapter 32

......................................................................

## Abiding in the Mind of Christ

*For who has known the mind of the Lord, that he will instruct Him? But we have the mind of Christ.*
*1 Corinthians 2:16*

It is so easy to look for hope from people, drugs, statistics or doctors. Joe's battle with cancer took me to a place of letting go of what I see. The internet is a great tool, but it became a source of discouragement. Melanoma does not have a whole lot of human hope. Most stories I read about people who had melanoma lived one to two years after diagnosis. I read dozens of clinical trials, but so many only added a few months to a person's life.

Cancer is a word that has a lot of power. I had to come to terms that it only had the power I gave it. Was it bigger than God? Every day, I give away power to things, people, and situations. I sometimes believe things I see more than what God says.

I realized my view of God tends to be fearful and mixed with lies about His character. Cancer forced me to see my concept of Him. My dialogue with Him was always truthful, but it seemed to be full of anger, almost like I had to get mad at Him to say what I really thought. He just wanted me to know the true Him.

I was basically forced to deal with God, as all the statistics, doctors, and stories had little hope. He was my last resort. His Word was either true or lies. I had to put my full hope in Him. I had to wait for Him to reveal Himself to me daily, and even moment by moment.

Words like grace, receive, believe, heal, love, friendship, wish, wait, look, knock, ask, all took on a different meaning when I saw them through a lens of love not fear.

1 John 4:18: *There is no fear in love; but perfect love casts out fear, because fear involves punishment, and the one who fears is not perfected in love.*

I needed to grow in knowing His love no matter what my circumstances looked like. I learned a few lessons here:

- If fear is creeping up inside of me, what lie is it telling me about God's character? Renounce that lie.

- If fear is creeping in, ask God to lead me out of it by giving me His Word to counter the lie I'm believing.

- If fear is creeping in, pray for deliverance from the thing I see. Ask to see His invisible help.

- If fear is creeping in, it will usually be telling me I am going to be punished (fear involves punishment). Believe that Jesus has taken that punishment on Himself. God's love language is grace.

So cancer's gift to me was "taking every thought captive" (2 Corinthians 10:5) to a God who loves me and died for me to prove it. I still do not catch on to the negative thoughts as fast as I wish. I still live with worry much longer than necessary. But I'm quicker to recognize there must be a lie robbing me of my loving God. He desires to lead me out of temptation especially the temptation that He is not loving and gracious, the temptation to believe in a false God.

I developed a daily (sometimes hourly) tool to help me catch these lies and renew my mind. The tool is **Renewing My Mind Slip** which can be found in the appendix of this book, and also in my book, *Dealing with Feelings, A Journal of God's Promises*, which is available on our website. This tool helps me stay or abide in God's love when all the lies of His character are coming at me.

## Chapter 33

· · · · · · · · · · · · · · · · · · · · · · · · · · · · · · · · · · · · · · · · · · · · · · · · · · · · · · · · · · · · · · · · · · · · ·

## Abiding in Losing All But Gaining Christ

*More than that, I count all things to be loss in view of the surpassing value of knowing Christ Jesus my Lord, for whom I have suffered the loss of all things, and count them but rubbish so that I may gain Christ . . . I press on toward the goal for the prize of the upward call of God in Christ Jesus.*
Philippians 3:8, 14

Somehow I think I can conquer the last battle of death by myself. I used to watch Oprah. She has had a few cancer patients on her show. They have written books on living life to the fullest each day, being grateful and positive, and of course, "in the moment."

All of that sounds great, but it is interesting that the question not asked is: "When you die, what do you think is going to happen to you?" I do not know how these people really feel about death. After facing death staring me in the face—I imagine most people begin to ask about the next life.

I've seen that most people answer the death question with "I've loved others, so I think I'll be okay." Yet how do we define love? If there is a God, it seems that He would define love for His creation. He would speak into His creation something about Himself that would reign true. Most of all, it seems that God would introduce *Himself* at some point into the eternal timeline of His creation. For me, He has introduced Jesus Christ. He is different from any other religious leader. He is the only one who said He *is* God. He did not just show us a way of life. He said, "I *am* the way, truth and life." Granted, saying and proving are quite different, but I'll go with the guy who said it and proved it by His Resurrection.

I need to let go of all I hold onto and count it as loss to gain Him and to know Him. Why? Because He is saying He is LIFE for now and for eternity.

Cancer has been a gift to me, not because it taught me how to live, but because it makes me face death. It gave me time to ask the hard questions, to seek God, to cry out to Him to make Himself real to me. If cancer just teaches us how to live this life, in my opinion it has missed its biggest call and purpose.

What is sadder is some people may not ask the most important questions because they are successful or feel they have lived a good life. Then they die in one afternoon from a freak accident. They did not believe on Jesus. They didn't think they needed a Savior. They were content and happy with their lives. They did not count all they had (or what they had done) as rubbish so that they could gain Christ and know the person who said, "I am the way, the truth, and the life" (John 14:6).

It seems to me counting all lost to gain Christ is the first step of really living and dying. I can say, our uninvited guest metastatic melanoma, helped me count my losses to know the living God.

Will I have more uninvited guests enter my home? Guests like failure, job losses, broken relationships or other illnesses? Probably. Will I want them to visit and stay long? No. Hopefully I will let God use them to clean out lies I have about Him and walk closer and deeper with His Son Jesus who is eternal life now.

One thing is certain: He has taken hold of me and I desire to take hold of that for which He has taken hold of me—His Son Jesus Christ.

# APPENDIX

. . . . . . . . . . . . . . . . . . . . . . . . . . . . . . . . . . . . . . . . . . . . . . . . . . . . . . . . . .

## An Abiding Tool for Renewing My Mind

*We are destroying speculations and every lofty thing raised up against the knowledge of God,
and we are taking every thought captive to the obedience of Christ.*
2 Corinthians 10:5

*For who has known the mind of the Lord, that he will instruct him? But we have the mind of Christ.*
1 Corinthians 2:16

Cancer helped me to learn to tap into "the mind of Christ" within me. The second verse above says we *already have* His mind. The first verse, 2 Corinthians 10:5, says God wants us to take every thought captive to Christ's obedience. I love that verse because it helped me not to depend on my obedience, my disciplined abilities, or my memory. I am to look away from myself and fix my mind not on *my* obedience, but "the obedience of Christ," or HIS obedience. I sometimes get so stressed that I am unable to memorize and meditate.

He gave me the promise of Joe's healing from John 15:7, *"If you abide in me and my words abide in you, ask whatever you wish, and it will be given you."* That verse was all about abiding in Him, which believers do from the new heart they have been given. Too many believers do not know they have a new heart that is united to Jesus' obedience. So many Christians are trying to get their own righteousness from their own devotion and their own obedience. Devotion and obedience becomes a very shaky foundation when one is sick and on strong medicines, or in pain physically or emotionally. Abiding for me was how I learned to walk more and more in faith in HIS Work in me. Looking to Jesus is so much more natural to me now. His love, His acceptance, His grace was the only place I could settle and stand.

I created this **Renewing My Mind Slip** which really worked for me to breakdown and process my struggles. I know this is not a new concept; however, I needed to take my thoughts captive on paper.

This is the process I have used and still use today, for myself; in support groups; and in one-on-one counseling..

# Renewing My Mind Slip

Situation: _____

_____

_____

_____

_____

Feelings: _____

_____

_____

_____

_____

Lies About God: _____

_____

_____

_____

_____

Flesh Actions: _____

_____

_____

_____

_____

Truth about God: _____

_____

_____

_____

_____

Spirit Action: _____

_____

_____

_____

_____

**How to fill out the slip:**

**Situation**: Identify daily anxieties and fears and write them down as a situation. I try to keep these short.

> Example: *I overheard a person say in the waiting room while Joe was in melanoma removal surgery that melanoma removal caused their relative's melanoma to spread even faster.*

**Feelings**: I then write down my feelings about this situation—facing them head on.

> Example: *Fearful, anxious, despondent, depressed; vulnerable that Joe will die and I'll be totally alone to provide for my two kids.*

**Lie About God**: Then I write the lie or lies about God that are at the root of those feelings.

> Example: *Anxiety and worry will stop God from fixing my problem.*

**Flesh actions**: Next I write out how I had acted in the "flesh," the old tendencies that rise up when I'm not trusting God.

> Example: *Obsessive thinking; over analyzing; overeating (I gained 30 pounds.)*

**Truth About Him**: I ask God to show me the truth about HIM, apart from what I am seeing. I love His Word for this, but He also used lots of ways to show me His goodness in practical ways.

> Example: *Matthew 6:25-27: For this reason I say to you, do not be worried about your life, as to what you will eat or what you will drink; nor for your body, as to what you will put on. Is not life more than food, and the body more than clothing? Look at the birds of the air, that they do not sow, nor reap nor gather into barns, and yet your heavenly Father feeds them. Are you not worth much more than they? Who of you by worrying can add a single hour to his life?*

**Spirit Action**: Finally, I ask Him for a "to-do" to move me into faith.

> Example: *Simply sitting and meditating on His love; being thankful for the moment I'm in; living in the NOW of God's love.*

It has been fun to see how God has used this **Renewing My Mind Slip** to start several ABIDING Groups, a part of Stronghold Ministry where we meet in small groups to learn how to abide together. Let me know if you'd like more info on how to start an Abiding Group. We've included several pages of **Renewing My Mind Slips** if you'd like to practice Abiding.

# Renewing My Mind Slip

Situation: _____

_____

_____

_____

_____

Feelings: _____

_____

_____

_____

_____

Lies About God: _____

_____

_____

_____

_____

Flesh Actions: _____

_____

_____

_____

_____

Truth about God: _____

_____

_____

_____

_____

Spirit Action: _____

_____

_____

_____

_____

# Renewing My Mind Slip

Situation: _____

_____

_____

_____

_____

Feelings: _____

_____

_____

_____

_____

Lies About God: _____

_____

_____

_____

Flesh Actions: _____

_____

_____

_____

Truth about God: _____

_____

_____

_____

Spirit Action: _____

_____

_____

_____

_____

# Renewing My Mind Slip

Situation: _____

_____

_____

_____

_____

Feelings: _____

_____

_____

_____

_____

Lies About God: _____

_____

_____

_____

_____

Flesh Actions: _____

_____

_____

_____

_____

Truth about God: _____

_____

_____

_____

_____

Spirit Action: _____

_____

_____

_____

_____

# Renewing My Mind Slip

**Situation:** _____
_____
_____
_____
_____

**Feelings:** _____
_____
_____
_____
_____

**Lies About God:** _____
_____
_____
_____
_____

**Flesh Actions:** _____
_____
_____
_____
_____

**Truth about God:** _____
_____
_____
_____
_____

**Spirit Action:** _____
_____
_____
_____
_____

# Renewing My Mind Slip

Situation: _____

_____

_____

_____

_____

Feelings: _____

_____

_____

_____

_____

Lies About God: _____

_____

_____

_____

_____

Flesh Actions: _____

_____

_____

_____

_____

Truth about God: _____

_____

_____

_____

_____

Spirit Action: _____

_____

_____

_____

_____

# Renewing My Mind Slip

Situation: _____

_____

_____

_____

_____

Feelings: _____

_____

_____

_____

_____

Lies About God: _____

_____

_____

_____

Flesh Actions: _____

_____

_____

_____

Truth about God: _____

_____

_____

_____

Spirit Action: _____

_____

_____

_____

# Renewing My Mind Slip

**Situation:** _____

_____

_____

_____

_____

**Feelings:** _____

_____

_____

_____

_____

**Lies About God:** _____

_____

_____

_____

_____

**Flesh Actions:** _____

_____

_____

_____

_____

**Truth about God:** _____

_____

_____

_____

_____

**Spirit Action:** _____

_____

_____

_____

_____

## Contact Information

. . . . . . . . . . . . . . . . . . . . . . . . . . . . . . . . . . . . . . . . . . . . . . . . . . . . . . . . . . . . . . . . .

### Website

www.mystronghold.org

### Email

tfor@mystronghold.org

### Phone

214-221-7007

### Joe and Terri Fornear's blog

www.mystronghold.org/blog/

### Mailing address

Stronghold Ministry
P.O. Box 38478
Dallas, TX 75238